# *Eat To Stay Healthy*

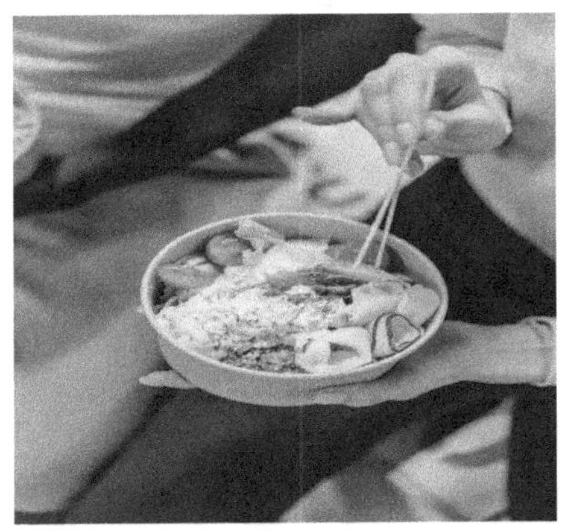

(Beating Diet with every Bite)

2024

**Clark Tyler**

# Table of contents

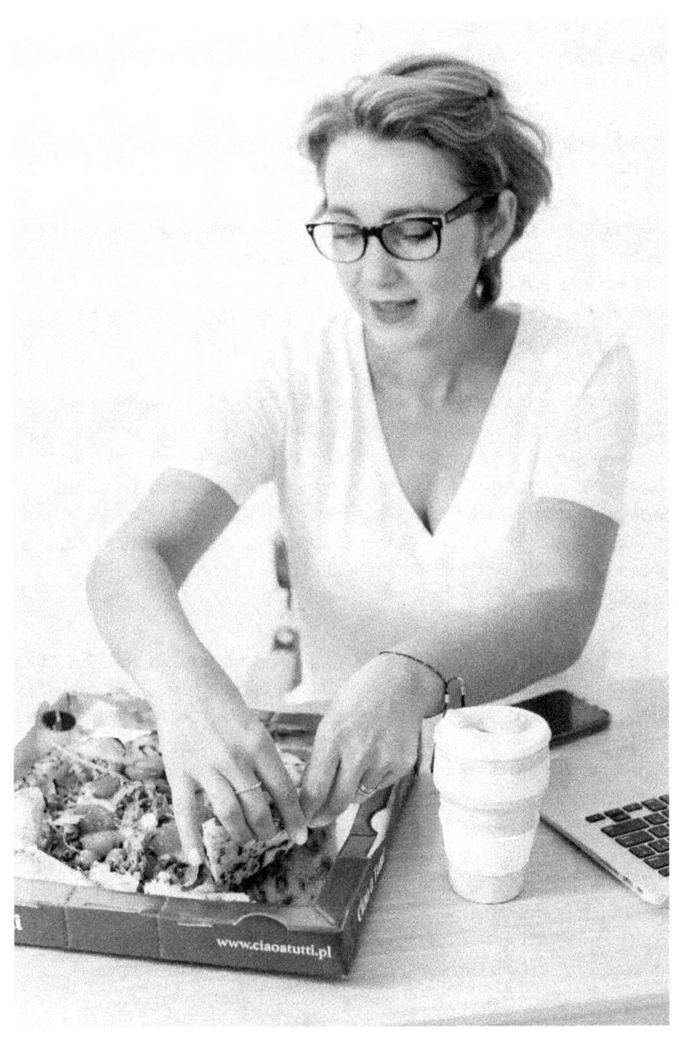

www.ciaoatutti.pl

# INTRODUCTION

A strange cook named Tricia lived in the busy city of Alma. She discovered the secret to long-lasting health one day while stirring a pot of colorful veggies. People from all across the city came to enjoy Tricia's famed culinary masterpieces. Her nutrient-dense foods filled the air with their perfume, and before long, the term "diet" became a celebration of flavor and vibrancy instead of something to be feared.

People's energy levels rose with each bite, leaving them feeling energized. In Tricia's small restaurant, friends gathered to share tales of their improved health brought on by her delicious recipes. The city adopted a wholistic approach to nutrition, and Tricia's motto, "Eat Healthy to Stay Healthy," was widely accepted.

Inspired by Tricia's experience, "Eat Healthy to Stay Healthy: Beating Diet with Every Bite" weaves together the happy victory over restrictive diets and the enchantment of mindful eating. Come along on this tasty journey to learn about the tasty route to wellbeing, as each chapter presents recipes that are a celebration of life as well as physical nourishment. With Alma, eating well is a joyful adventure rather than a scary goal, and each mouthful is a step toward conquering the traditional diet.

Sustaining a nutritious diet is essential for general health. Essential nutrients are provided by a proper diet, supporting bodily processes. A healthy diet boosts immunity and lowers vulnerability to disease. It helps control weight, reducing the chance of obesity-related illnesses like diabetes and heart problems. Foods high in nutrients support healthy brain function, improving mood and cognitive function. Eating a healthy diet promotes effective digestion and helps to avoid digestive problems. It encourages robust muscles and bones, which support physical activity and guard against injury. A healthy diet also has a favorable effect on skin health and promotes a glowing complexion. Maintaining good eating practices over time lowers the chance of developing chronic illnesses, resulting in a longer, more active life.

CHAPTER ONE

## 1.1 IMPORTANCE OF HEALTHY EATING

1. Nutrient Adequacy: Eating a healthy diet guarantees that vital nutrients, such as vitamins, minerals, proteins, and carbs, are consumed, which enhances general wellbeing. These nutrients are essential for many body processes, including immune system maintenance, growth, and preserving good health.

2. Disease Prevention: Heart disease, diabetes, and some types of cancer can all be avoided with a balanced diet. Include a range of fruits, vegetables, whole grains, and lean meats in your diet to give your body the nutrition it needs to ward off potential health hazards.

3. Weight Management: By encouraging a balanced calorie intake, healthy eating helps with weight control. Nutrient-dense diets and portion control help people reach and maintain a healthy weight, which lowers their risk of problems from obesity.

4. Energy Boost: A healthy diet gives your body the energy it requires to carry out daily tasks. A diet rich in complex carbs and sufficient protein that is well-balanced raises energy levels over time and improves general health and productivity.

5. Mental Health: Foods high in nutrients promote mental and cognitive health. For example, omega-3 fatty acids from fish have been associated with happier moods, while antioxidants from fruits and vegetables may help maintain cognitive function.

6. Digestive Health: Foods high in fiber, like fruits, vegetables, and whole grains, facilitate digestion and help avoid constipation. Effective food absorption and waste removal are made possible by a healthy digestive tract, which also supports gastrointestinal health generally.

## 1.2 Goals of the book

1. Inform Readers on Nutritional Fundamentals: Give them a thorough grasp of the important nutrients, where they come from, and how they affect general health.

2. Develop Balanced Meal Plans: Provide doable meal plans that highlight a diet that is well-rounded and incorporates a range of food groups to satisfy dietary requirements.

3. Encourage Mindful Eating Practices: Tell readers to relish every bite, be mindful of hunger and fullness cues, and be present during meals.

4. Emphasize Nutrient-Rich Ingredients and Superfoods: Present a variety of foods that are high in antioxidants, vitamins, and minerals to enable readers to make wise dietary decisions.

5. Dispel Often Held Myths About Diets: Dispel myths around diets and provide information on evidence-based methods for maintaining a balanced diet.

6. Provide Easy and Healthful Recipes: To make healthy eating accessible and pleasurable, offer simple-to-follow recipes that suit a variety of palates and dietary needs.

7. Put a Focus on Sustainable Eating: Examine how food choices affect the environment and encourage sustainable lifestyles that are good for the environment and human health.

8. Promote Frequent Physical Activity: Highlight the significance of integrating exercise into a healthy lifestyle, enhancing the dietary recommendations with a comprehensive outlook on wellbeing.

9. Provide Dining Out Strategies: Give readers advice on how to choose healthily when dining out and how to keep a balanced diet even in social situations.

10. Offer Tools for Long-Term Success: Give readers the resources they need to keep up a healthy lifestyle, including how to set reasonable objectives, monitor their progress, and overcome obstacles in their path to improved health.

CHAPTER TWO

## 2.1 What is Fitness and Nutrition

Fitness reflects a person's capacity to handle the rigors of everyday life and includes both physical and mental well-being. Strength, flexibility, cardiovascular endurance, and body composition are all involved. A balanced strategy that includes regular exercise, a healthy diet, and enough sleep is necessary to achieve fitness. It is a comprehensive condition of health that promotes the best possible physical and mental performance rather than just the absence of disease. Fitness is dynamic; it changes with age and with changing habits. Frequent exercise strengthens muscles, strengthens the heart, and increases mental toughness. In the end, it's a lifelong adventure that highlights the significance of continuing to lead an active, healthy lifestyle.

The process by which organisms acquire and use nutrients for development, energy, and the upkeep of physiological processes is known as nutrition. It entails consuming vital components through food, including proteins, lipids, carbs, vitamins, and minerals. These nutrients are essential for maintaining metabolism, forming tissues, and controlling a number of physiological activities. For optimum health, a balanced diet is essential since it provides the building blocks needed for many body processes. Malnutrition, inadequacies, and a host of other health problems can result from poor nutrition. In order to prevent nutritional imbalances and promote general well-being, it is essential to understand nutritional needs and make educated food choices.

## 2.2. Symbiotic Relationship

A person's overall health depends on their diet and level of fitness. The body gets its fuel from a healthy diet, which supplies the vital vitamins, minerals, and energy required for exercise. On the other hand, consistent exercise increases muscular growth, speeds up metabolism, and raises fitness levels all around. Their dynamic relationship optimizes cardiovascular health, emotional well-being, and weight management. The efficacy of one can be hampered by neglecting another. A balanced diet and regular exercise create a synergistic environment that supports a stronger, healthier body. This is how they work together harmoniously.

## 2.2 **Exercise Routines**

It takes a balanced approach to exercise and nutrition to reach overall fitness. Mix up your program by including cardiovascular, strength, and flexibility activities. Start at least five days a week with 30 minutes of moderate-intensity cardio, such as brisk walking or cycling. Two to three times a week, perform strength training exercises that focus on your primary muscle groups, such as lunges, push-ups, and squats. Make flexibility a priority by engaging in dynamic stretching or yoga to improve joint mobility and lower the chance of injury. As your fitness increases, progressively increase the intensity and duration of your workouts. Incorporate enjoyable activities into the routine to make it enduring. Adopt a well-rounded diet that is high in whole grains, fruits, vegetables, lean proteins, and healthy fats. Set water intake as a top priority and monitor meal sizes to limit caloric intake. Reduce your intake of sugar-filled beverages, processed meals, and alcohol. To receive individualized advice, think about speaking with a nutritionist. Recall that consistency is essential. For long-term well-being, track your progress, make any adjustments to your routine, and adopt a holistic approach to nutrition and training.

## 2.3 **Meal Planning**

A balance of macronutrients and micronutrients can be found in a well-rounded meal plan that supports nutrition and exercise.

Start with a protein-rich food, such as fish, tofu, or grilled chicken, which provides the necessary amino acids for muscle growth and repair. Combine this with complex carbs like brown rice, sweet potatoes, or quinoa to keep your energy levels up. Include a range of vibrant veggies, such as bell peppers, spinach, and broccoli, to guarantee a spectrum of minerals and vitamins. To promote general health and satiety, include healthy fats from foods like avocados, almonds, and olive oil. For consistent energy throughout the day, choose smaller, more frequent meals. For a protein and antioxidant boost, pair Greek yogurt with berries or almonds as a snack. Consistently drink water to stay hydrated, especially before and after workouts. To replace glycogen levels and promote healing, try having a shake with whey protein and a banana after your workout. Cut back on processed foods, sugary snacks, and too much coffee. Adjust serving sizes based on personal requirements, taking activity levels and fitness objectives into account.

CHAPTER THREE

## 3.1. **Healthy Eating on Budget**

Making economical and wise decisions when it comes to eating well requires preparing ahead. Invest in reasonably priced staples that are high in fiber, protein, and complex carbs, such as brown rice, lentils, and beans. Select a selection of frozen veggies to guarantee a range of nutrients. Frozen vegetables are affordable and retain their nutritious content. When it's feasible, buy in bulk to save money over time.

Cheap sources of protein are yogurt, eggs, and tuna in cans. Buy seasonal produce while it's on sale since it's usually more affordable and has the highest nutritional value. To maximize ingredients and reduce food waste, plan your meals in advance. Think about generic or store brands, which are frequently less expensive without compromising quality.

Compared to eating out, cooking at home usually costs less since you can manage the products and serving sizes. Accept components that may be utilized for both breakfast and snacks, such as oats. Go online for inexpensive meal ideas and try different combinations of spices to enhance taste without breaking the bank. Give whole foods a higher priority than processed ones, as they frequently provide more nutrients for the same price. A healthy diet may be maintained on a tight budget with careful planning and inventiveness.

## 3.2 **Affordable nutrient-rich Foods**

Some examples of affordable nutrient-rich Foods that will help you stay fit and diet filled without needing to break the bank:

| Category | Food | Nutrients Highlights |
| --- | --- | --- |
| Proteins | Eggs | High-grade protein, necessary amino acids |

| | Canned Tuna | Lean protein, omega-3 fatty acids |
| --- | --- | --- |
| | Lentils | Plant-based protein, fiber, iron |
| | Greek Yogurt | Protein, probiotics, calcium |
| Whole Grains | Brown Rice | Complex carbohydrates, fiber |
| | Oats | Fiber, manganese, whole grain goodness |
| | Whole Wheat PastaFiber, | Fiber, B-vitamins |
| Fruits | Bananas | Potassium, vitamins, natural sweetness |
| | Apples | Fiber, antioxidants |
| | Oranges | Vitamin C, fiber |
| Vegetables | Carrots | Beta-carotene, vitamins |
| | Spinach | Iron, vitamins, antioxidants |
| | Broccoli | Vitamin C, fiber, folate |
| Healthy Fats | Avocados | Monounsaturated fats, |

| | | |
|---|---|---|
| | | potassium |
| | Olive Oil | Monounsaturated fats, antioxidants |
| | | |

These reasonably priced, nutrient-dense foods offer a wide variety of vital elements that are necessary for a well-balanced diet.

### 3.3 **Shopping tips for Groceries**

1. Plan meals ahead to prepare a precise grocery list.

2. For selections that are high in nutrients, give fresh fruits and vegetables priority.

3. Pick fish, poultry, and beans as your lean protein sources.

4. Choose whole grains for extra fiber instead than processed ones.

5. To get different kinds of nutrients, including a range of vibrant fruit.

Look for fresh and lightly processed products along the store's perimeter.

7. Check the nutrition facts on food labels to make well-informed decisions.

8. To encourage a better diet, limit processed and sugary snacks.

9. Save money on necessities like grains and beans by purchasing in bulk.

10. When you go shopping, don't forget to pack water and herbal teas.

11. Use nuts and avocados as a source of healthful fat.

12. To increase your calcium intake, use dairy products with reduced fat or dairy substitutes.

13. Don't shop when hungry to avoid impulse purchases of unhealthy foods.

14. To add taste without adding too many calories, try experimenting with different herbs and spices.

15. When choosing convenience above nutrition, go for frozen fruits and vegetables.

16. Be aware of portion sizes when purchasing packaged goods.

17. Add foods like fatty fish or flaxseeds that are high in omega-3 fatty acids.

18. For improved freshness and cost-effectiveness, think about purchasing in-season food.

19. Avoid using processed sweets and use natural sweeteners like honey or maple syrup.

20. To cut costs on healthy selections, keep an eye out for deals and discounts.

## 3.4 **Mindful Eating Practice**

Eating mindfully is a discipline that promotes experiencing every moment of the meal, developing a stronger bond with food, and enhancing general wellbeing. It entails using all of one's senses, living in the present, and savoring every meal without passing judgment.

When eating mindfully, people concentrate on the flavors, textures, and colors of their meal. They chew slowly and take pleasure in every bite, appreciating the experience of eating. A mindful eater also discerns between physical and emotional hunger by paying attention to their body's signals of fullness and hunger.

Instances of attentive eating consist of:

1. Sensory Awareness: Engaging senses by examining the scent, taste, and texture of each mouthful, enriching the dining experience.

2. Chewing mindfully: Chewing slowly and allowing the body to tell you when it's full can help you avoid overindulging.

3. Appreciating Food Origins: Fostering gratitude and a closer bond with meals by considering the path that food takes from source to plate.

4. Listening to Hunger Cues: Recognizing when hunger comes and distinguishing between emotional and physical hunger, making educated decisions about when and what to eat.

5. Eating with Intention: Taking use of meals to their fullest potential by savoring the sustenance without interruptions from devices or work.

In general, mindful eating promotes a better approach to feeding by encouraging a more aware and pleasant conception.

CHAPTER FOUR

## 4.1 Unique Dietary consideration

Particular food requirements arise from ethical decisions, cultural customs, and personal health requirements. Managing health-related issues might include dietary alterations needed for illnesses like diabetes, allergies, or intolerances. Global cultural dietary preferences differ, impacting decisions based on customs, religious convictions, or the accessibility of particular foods in a given area. People may be motivated by ethical concerns to adopt vegetarianism, veganism, or other specialized diets in order to minimize their environmental impact and conform to their own personal ideals. Comprehending distinct dietary requirements is essential for advancing general health and honoring a range of viewpoints. In order to provide a holistic approach to food intake that takes into account each person's individuality, it entails adjusting dietary choices to take health, cultural background, and ethical beliefs into consideration.

## 4.2 Accommodating Dietary limitations

In order to properly meet dietary restrictions, a careful and thorough approach must be taken. Start by getting a complete grasp of each person's unique dietary needs or limits, taking into account any allergies, intolerances, or lifestyle preferences. This information is the basis for developing a varied and inclusive meal that meets a range of requirements. Provide a variety of options when organizing meals, making sure to account for frequent allergies or dietary constraints. Dishes should have clear labels that include pertinent information about ingredients and any allergies. This builds trust and gives people the capacity to make educated decisions. Have frank discussions with those who have food restrictions. Invite them to express their choices and be open to suggestions. This cooperative strategy shows a dedication to attending to each person's needs while also guaranteeing inclusion. To ensure correct ingredient handling and avoid cross-contamination, kitchen staff training is essential. This attention to detail emphasizes the value of preserving the integrity of specialty foods from preparation to presentation and goes beyond the kitchen to the complete dining experience. Menus should be updated often to take into account shifting dietary trends and seasonal items. Providing everyone with a dynamic dining experience requires creativity and flexibility. A smooth and enriching component of culinary offerings is made possible by embracing adaptation, a dedication to diversity, and upholding open lines of communication.

## 4.3 **Plant - Based Vegan Diets**

Plant-based vegan diets emphasize eating only plant-based meals and avoiding all animal products. This dietary option provides vital elements, including fiber, vitamins, and minerals, by emphasizing fruits, vegetables, grains, legumes, nuts, and seeds. Diets based mostly on plants are frequently linked to a host of health advantages, such as decreased risks of heart disease, hypertension, and several types of cancer. Going vegan for health reasons is not the only benefit to the environment. The raising of livestock has a major negative impact on water pollution, greenhouse gas emissions, and deforestation. People may address climate change issues and lessen their ecological impact by opting for plant-based alternatives. This helps with conservation efforts. Plant-based veganism places a high value on ethical issues. Many people choose this way of living in order to live up to the ideals of kindness and non-violence toward animals. People try to lessen the pain that animals endure as a result of industrial farming and slaughterhouse methods by abstaining from animal products. To sum up, plant-based vegan diets promote a lifestyle that aims to improve human well-being, the environment, and animal welfare by providing a comprehensive approach to health, environmental sustainability, and ethical issues.

## 4.4 **Gluten and Allergen free option**

A gluten- and allergen-free diet is designed to accommodate those who are sensitive to gluten or who have allergies to certain types of wheat, barley, rye, and their derivatives. Some people may react adversely to gluten, a composite protein, resulting in stomach discomfort or more severe symptoms. Gluten-free alternatives include grains like rice, quinoa, and maize to offer a healthy substitute while maintaining a broad nutritional profile. Additionally, an allergen-free diet goes beyond gluten to accommodate those with a variety of sensitivities. This means staying away from common allergens, including dairy, soy, nuts, and shellfish. By doing this, people can lessen their chance of experiencing allergic reactions, which can range from minor discomfort to serious reactions like anaphylaxis. Whole, unprocessed foods, including fruits, vegetables, lean meats, and gluten-free grains, are prioritized in a balanced gluten- and allergen-free diet. In the process, possible triggers are avoided, and nutritional adequacy is promoted. Because manufactured goods may include hidden sources of gluten and allergies, it becomes imperative to carefully read labels. All things considered, following a gluten- and allergen-free diet necessitates making well-informed food selections, closely examining ingredients, and devotedly preserving a balanced, allergen-safe nutritional profile.

CHAPTER FIVE

## 5.1 Overcoming obstacles

When dieting, overcoming setbacks and upholding good habits calls for a calculated strategy. First, in order to prevent feeling overwhelmed, set reasonable and attainable goals and make small, incremental adjustments. To guarantee sufficient sustenance, develop a meal plan that is sustainable and well-balanced, encompassing a range of nutrient-rich foods. Building a solid support network may be very important. Talk about your objectives with loved ones or friends who can support and empathize. Seek expert advice from dietitians or associate with like-minded individuals to build a feeling of accountability. To stop emotional eating, identify different coping strategies for emotional triggers. A better relationship with food may be fostered by mindful eating, which involves enjoying every meal and paying attention to hunger signs. To prevent making snap decisions, have a plan and prepare meals in advance. Store wholesome snacks close at hand to lessen the temptation to go for junk food. Recognize progress, celebrate little successes, and maintain your motivation. Finally, rather than seeing setbacks as failures, see them as teaching opportunities. If necessary, modify your goals and carry on with resilience. Overcoming challenges and promoting a long-term, healthy diet may be accomplished by fusing realistic tactics with an optimistic outlook.

## 5.2 Long-term Methods for Success

Adopting sustainable strategies is necessary to maintain healthy eating habits over the long run. First and foremost, prioritize a diet that is balanced and includes a range of fruits, vegetables, complete grains, and lean meats. Make a livable meal plan that will fit into your schedule and be simpler to follow with time. Pay attention to your body's signals of hunger and fullness to cultivate mindful eating habits. Instead of focusing on restrictive diets, stress moderation, and portion management, Make small, lasting improvements to your diet by starting with small adjustments. Celebrate your successes with food and stop seeing occasional indulgences as a sign of weakness to build a healthy relationship with it. In addition to a nutritious diet, regular physical activity enhances general wellbeing. Seek expert help when necessary, involve friends and family in your journey, and surround yourself with encouraging people. Routines encourage consistency, which makes it simpler to stick to good behaviors. Maintain current knowledge of advancements in the area, and never stop learning about nutrition and wellbeing. Finally, keep in mind that eating a nutritious diet is a lifelong process.

CHAPTER SIX

6.1 Boost Breakfast

A high-nutrient breakfast is an essential part of your daily diet and is critical to your overall health. In order to enhance energy levels, cognitive function, and general health, start your day with a balanced combination of macronutrients and micronutrients. Add nutritious grains, such as quinoa or oats, which are rich in complex carbs that release energy over time. Add foods high in lean protein, such as almonds, Greek yogurt, or eggs, to help with satiety and muscle regeneration. Use a range of vibrant fruits and vegetables to receive your fill of vital vitamins, minerals, and antioxidants. Leafy greens, citrus fruits, and berries are great options. Good fats from foods like olive oil, avocados, and nuts support a healthy brain and facilitate the absorption of nutrients. As alternatives to dairy products, think of plant-based or calcium-rich foods. Drink water or herbal tea with your meal, since staying hydrated is important. Reduce processed meals and added sugars to maximize nutritional value. Breakfast provides a powerful nutritional boost that supports general well-being and sustains energy for everyday activities, laying a solid foundation for the day.

## 6.2 **Lunch Dynamo concept**

The Lunch Dynamo idea emphasizes a healthy, balanced midday meal to improve general health by incorporating a wellness formula into dietary practices. This method acknowledges lunch as an essential part of maintaining energy levels and fostering well being all day long.

For instance, including a range of nutrient-dense foods—like whole grains, lean meats, and vibrant vegetables—supplies vital vitamins and minerals. A well-planned lunch maintains physical energy, improves cognitive performance, and helps with weight control.

Imagine quinoa, grilled chicken breast, and a colorful selection of veggies for lunch. This blend provides complex carbs for long-term energy, proteins for muscle repair, and a variety of vitamins and antioxidants. Such a meal supports the immune system and helps prevent sickness, in addition to providing the body with nourishment.

In addition, the Lunch Dynamo concept's mindful eating techniques include appreciating every mouthful, boosting digestive health, and developing a good relationship with food. This all-encompassing strategy guarantees that lunch turns into a vital component of sustaining a healthy lifestyle, establishing a dynamic balance for general wellbeing.

## 6.3 **Healthful Dinner Delights**

A nutritious dinner The goal of the Delights in Wellness formula is to offer a healthy, well-balanced eating experience. The cornerstone is using an array of nutrient-dense components that support general health. Fish and grilled chicken are examples of lean proteins that support fullness and healthy muscles. Complex carbohydrates are found in whole grains like brown rice and quinoa, which provide long-lasting energy.

Sufficient amounts of vibrant veggies guarantee a range of vitamins and minerals essential for internal processes. Good fats, found in foods like avocados and olive oil, support the health of the heart and the absorption of nutrients. Proper portion proportions support a healthy lifestyle by helping with weight management.

To maintain nutritional integrity, the preparation method places a strong emphasis on minimum processing. Seasonings are picked for their possible health advantages as well as to improve flavor. The result is a gastronomic adventure that not only pleases palates but also promotes general health by offering vital nutrients without adding harmful ingredients or extra calories. Healthy Dinner Delights is a thoughtful alternative for anybody looking for a nutritious and wholesome dinner option since it adheres to the principles of balanced nutrition.

### Overview of Core Principles

"Eat to Stay Healthy: Beating Diet with Every Bite" offers a thorough analysis of nutrition with a focus on fundamental ideas that support long-term health. The book emphasizes the value of eating a balanced diet and advises against following restrictive diets. It encourages readers to follow their bodies' cues and promotes a thoughtful and intuitive eating style. In his exploration of the importance of nutrient-dense, whole foods, the author highlights the role that fruits, vegetables, lean meats, and whole grains play in preserving optimum health. The fundamental ideas of the book promote a holistic understanding of nutrition that takes into account both physical and mental elements, placing an emphasis on food quality rather than calorie tracking. Moreover, "Eat to Stay Healthy" incorporates scientific discoveries into easily understood content, enabling readers to make knowledgeable decisions. The book promotes customized eating plans, acknowledging that every person has different needs. It also discusses the importance of maintaining hydration, the influence of lifestyle choices on general health, and mindful eating practices. The main ideas presented in this book are about enabling readers to make decisions that will ultimately promote their long-term health and well-being, dispelling diet misconceptions, and encouraging a positive and sustainable connection with food.

Encouragement

Adopting a better lifestyle by following "Eat to Stay Healthy" is a journey of transformation that goes beyond simple nutrition. This energizing method of eating encourages you to enjoy each mouthful with the intention of feeding your body and spirit. The fundamental idea is straightforward yet profound: eat foods that support your health and create inner vibrancy. Keep in mind that moderation is essential in your pursuit of a healthier lifestyle. "Eat to Stay Healthy" invites you to celebrate the colorful palette that nature gives by indulging in a wide variety of nutrient-rich meals. Savor the freshness of fresh fruits, crunchy veggies, lean meats, and healthy grains—a harmonious combination of tastes that not only satisfies your hunger but also provides your body with vital nutrients. This is a journey about abundance in the healthiest sense, not deprivation. Give yourself permission to enjoy trying out new, healthful dishes that support your wellness objectives. Appreciate the good things you do every day, and remember to celebrate progress rather than perfection. "Eat to Stay Healthy" encourages conscious eating by raising awareness of the physical and emotional effects of food. Imagine, as you start along this route, living a life in which every meal is a step toward a better, more vibrant version of yourself and in which your decisions empower you. Accept the knowledge in these pages, relish the process of developing a good relationship with food, and bask in the glory of a life well lived by the decisions you make about what to eat and how to remain well.

Conclusion

As the last pages of "Eat to Stay Healthy" flipped, Tricia thought back on her path of transformation that was aided by the knowledge included in each chapter of the book. The story threaded through the complexities of nutrition, revealing the significant influence of mindful eating on general health. The book had given her the confidence to make knowledgeable dietary decisions by providing her with colorful examples and knowledgeable insights into the complex link between food and health. The last chapter acted as a guide, stressing the value of balance and sustainable practices. With a fresh understanding of the significant influence of mindful diet and equipped with useful knowledge, Tricia concluded the book with a renewed resolve to nourish her body and mind. The last words didn't mean the end of the voyage; rather, they signaled the beginning of a new chapter in Tricia's life, one in which the ideas behind "Eat to Stay Healthy" served as the cornerstone for a healthy and fulfilling future.